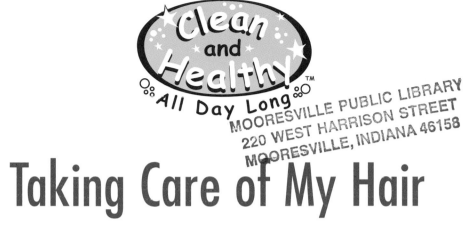

PowerKids Readers:

Clean and Healthy All Day Long™

Taking Care of My Hair

Elizabeth Vogel

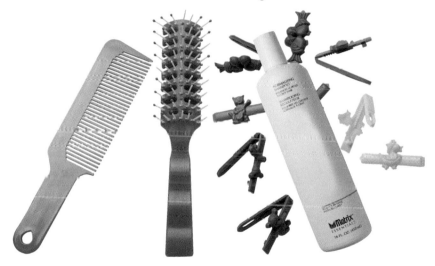

The Rosen Publishing Group's
PowerKids Press™
New York

1

Published in 2001 by The Rosen Publishing Group, Inc.
29 East 21st Street, New York, NY 10010

First Edition

Book Design: Danielle Primiceri
Layout: Felicity Erwin

Photo Illustrations by Thaddeus Harden

Vogel, Elizabeth.
   Taking care of my hair / by Elizabeth Vogel.
      p. cm. — (PowerKids Readers clean and healthy all day long)
   Includes index.
   Summary: Describes how to take care of one's hair so that it will be healthy.
   ISBN: 0-8239-5685-7 (lib. bdg. : alk. paper)
      1. Hair—Care and hygiene—Juvenile literature. [1. Hair—Care and hygiene.]
I. Title. II. Series.

RL91 .V644 2000
646.7'24—dc21
                                                          99-055188

Manufactured in the United States of America

Contents

Hair needs a lot of care.
I brush my hair to keep it
soft and healthy.

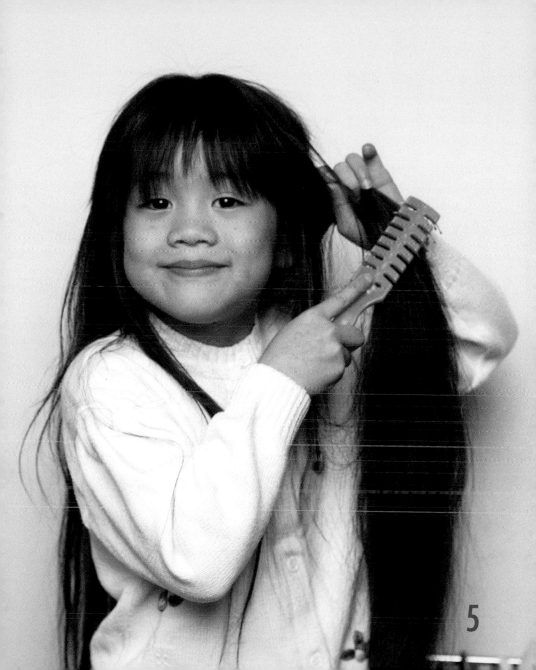

5

I have long hair. Hair can be long or short, straight or curly.

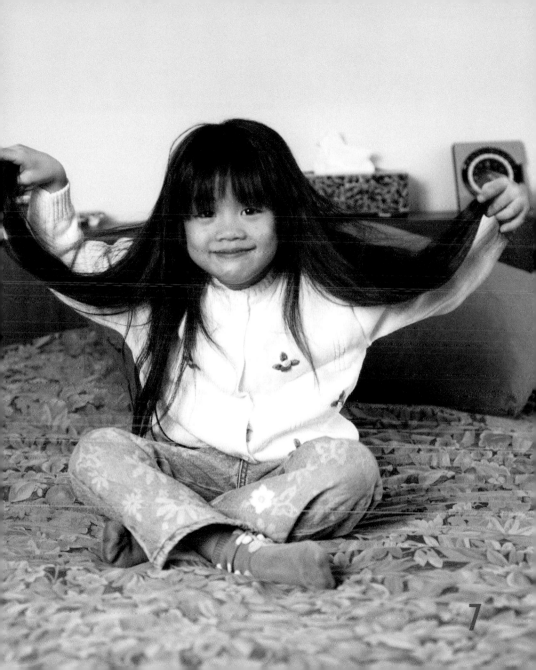

Sometimes I wear barrettes in my hair. Barrettes keep my hair neat.

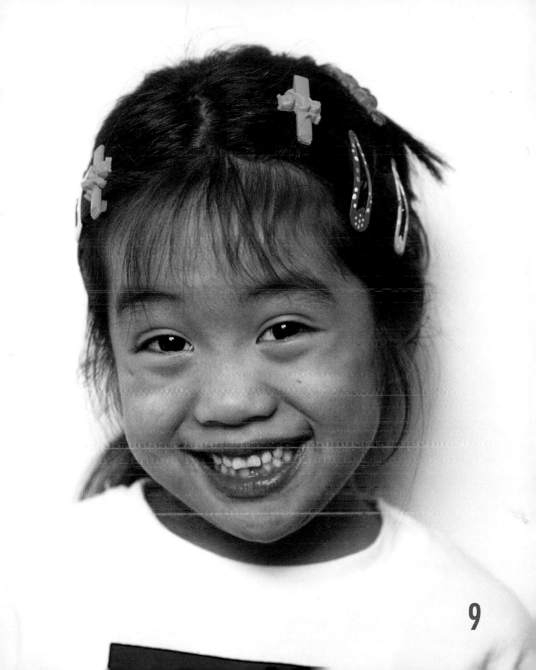

9

Sometimes I wear my hair down. It is fun to wear my hair different ways.

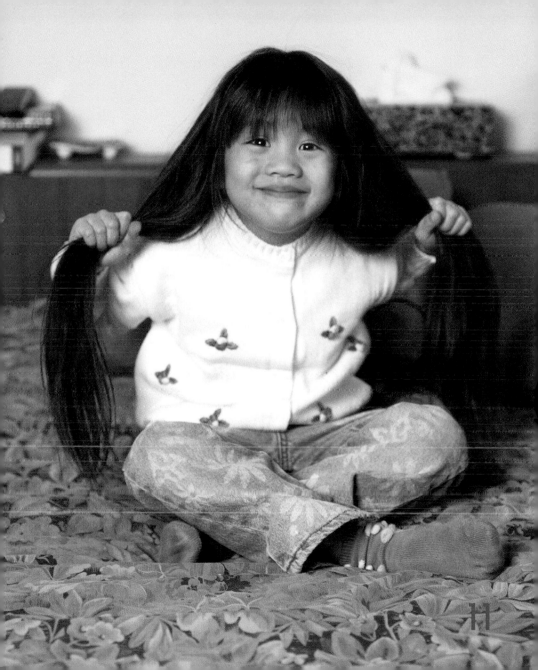

Healthy hair grows six inches each year. I go to the hairdresser to get my hair cut. Haircuts keep my hair healthy.

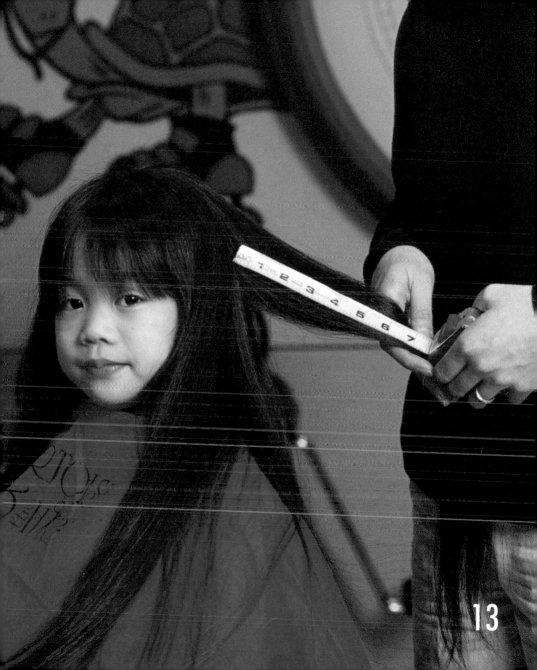

Every type of hair needs to be cut. The hairdresser uses scissors to cut my hair.

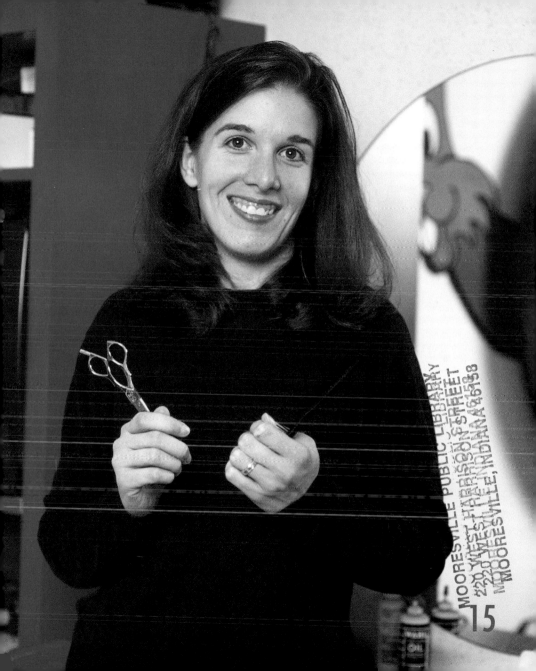

15

First the hairdresser washes my hair. She uses shampoo. Shampoo washes the dirt out of my hair.

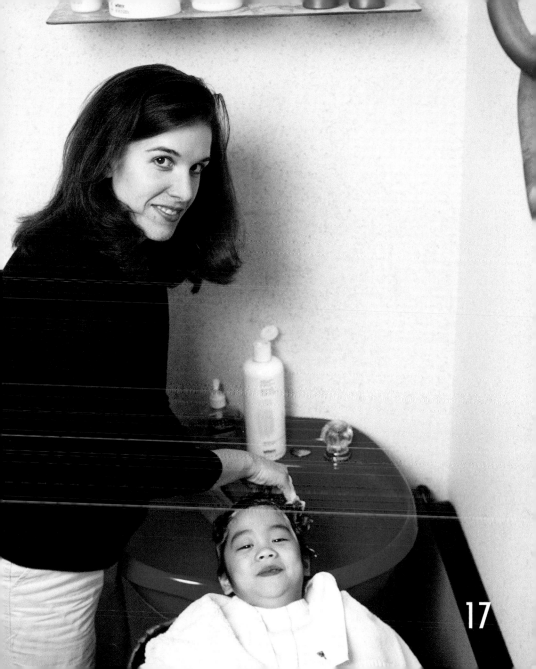

17

Then the hairdresser rinses the shampoo out of my hair. She makes sure all the soapy bubbles are gone.

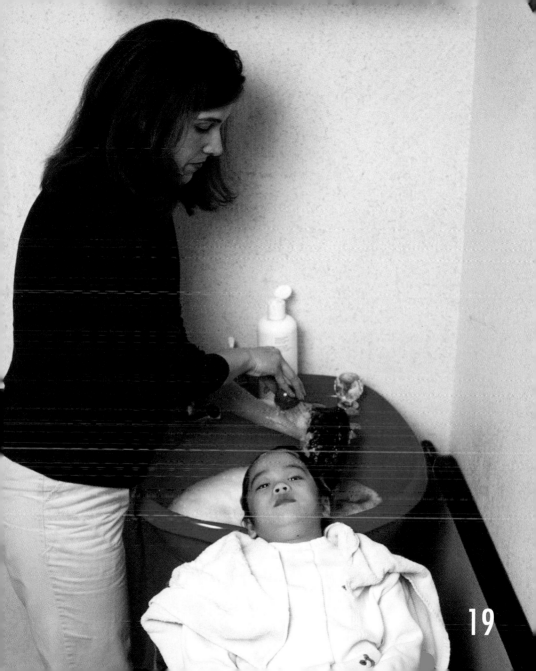

I wash my hair at home, too. I use a comb when my hair is wet. Combing my hair helps to keep tangles out. I love to take care of my clean and healthy hair!

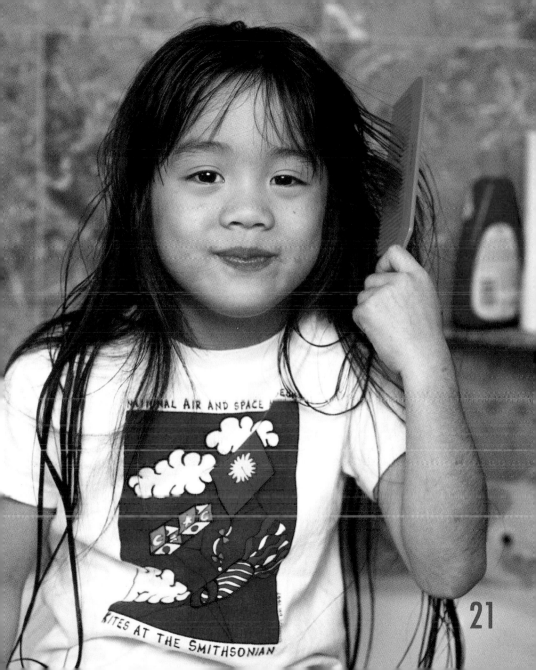

21

Words to Know

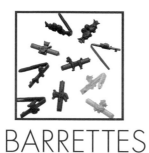 BARRETTES

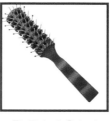 BRUSH

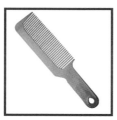 COMB

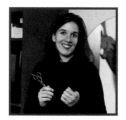 HAIRDRESSER

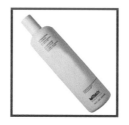 SHAMPOO

Here are more books to read about taking care of your hair:

My Hair Is Beautiful: Because It Is Mine
By Paula Dejoie
Writers & Readers Publishing, Inc.

Will Gets a Haircut
By Olaf Landstrom, Lena Landstrom
R & S Books

To learn more about taking care of your hair, check out this Web site:
www.headlice.org/kids/headgames/hairforce/hairforce.htm

Index

Word Count: 165

Note to Parents, Teachers, and Librarians

PowerKids Readers are specially designed to get emergent and beginning readers excited about learning to read. Simple stories and concepts are paired with photographs of real kids in real-life situations. Spirited characters and story lines that kids can relate to help readers respond to written language by linking meaning with their own everyday experiences. Sentences are short and simple, employing a basic vocabulary of sight words, as well as new words that describe familiar things and places. Large type, clean design, and photographs corresponding directly to the text all help children to decipher meaning. Features such as a picture glossary and an index help children get the most out of PowerKids Readers. Lists of related books and Web sites encourage kids to explore other sources and to continue the process of learning. With their engaging stories and vivid photo-illustrations, PowerKids Readers inspire children with the interest and confidence to return to these books again and again. It is this rich and rewarding experience of success with language that gives children the opportunity to develop a love of reading and learning that they will carry with them throughout their lives.